GET YOUR BIGGEST QUESTIONS ANSWERED

WHAT SHOULD I EAT?

WHICH SUPPLEMENTS SHOULD I TAKE?

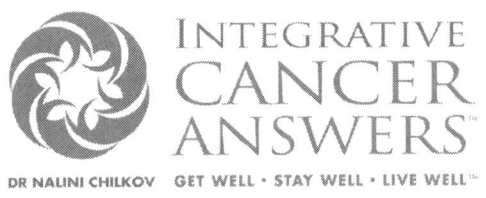

Copyright © 2014-2015 by Integrative Cancer Answers
All rights reserved.

No part of this book may be reproduced in any form or by any electronic or mechanical means including information storage and retrieval systems, without permission in writing from the author. The only exception is by a reviewer, who may quote short excerpts in a review.

Disclaimer

The information herein and on our websites is provided for informational purposes only. The information is a result of years of practice experience by the author. This information is not intended as a substitute for the advice provided by your physician or other healthcare professional or any information contained on or in any product label or packaging.

Do not use the information herein or on our websites for diagnosing or treating a health problem or disease, or prescribing medication or other treatment. Always speak with your physician or other healthcare professional before taking any medication or nutritional, herbal or homeopathic supplement, or using any treatment for a health problem.

If you have or suspect that you have a medical problem, contact your health care provider promptly. Do not disregard professional medical advice or delay in seeking professional advice because of something you have read herein or on our web site.

Information provided herein and on our websites and the use of any products or services purchased from our websites by you DOES NOT create a doctor-patient relationship between you and any of the physicians affiliated with our web sites.

Information and statements regarding dietary supplements have not been evaluated by the Food and Drug Administration and are not intended to diagnose, treat, cure, or prevent any disease.

Praise for Dr. Nalini and Integrative Cancer Answers

Last year I almost died of advanced cancer. Nobody should have to go through what I experienced - My doctors are amazed. After only two weeks of starting my nutritional supplements, herbal medicines, morning smoothie and cancer fighting diet, my health and vitality doubled and in three months, I'm feeling close to 100% - Dr. Nalini Chilkov is my secret weapon for perfect health – she's practical, pragmatic and brilliant.
Mike Koenigs
Advanced Colorectal Cancer
Best Selling Author and Speaker

Finally, someone who is looking at the whole and long term picture; not just deploying nuclear bombs in my body and waiting to see the results. Now I feel like I can be pro-active in my battle and not just a vessel for harmful but necessary chemicals. So much of her nutritional advice, as my husband is a wonderful and informed cook, was on our radar but thanks to Dr. Chilkov, we now have the needed impetus to clean up those last nasty eating choices. Her encouragement to use this illness to create life changing habits was empowering and the comfort of knowing that she will be in my corner for a long time to come is a huge emotional boost. Even the process of sorting through the plethora of vitamin/supplement bottles feels liberating and the acupuncture session was a definite boost to my energy level & well being. I cannot thank you enough for your all knowing kindness. With extreme gratitude for giving a life changing gift. I am not sure where to begin to thank you. My meeting with Dr. Chilkov was the most needed of medicines.
J.C., Advanced Ovarian Cancer Patient

Her skill has helped me to heal physically. More importantly, her compassion and patience helped me to grow and develop as a human being. Rarely in life do you meet someone who wondrously heals and teaches. In so doing, they expand and change your life. Nalini is one of those rare people.
M.B., 21st Century Funds

You have treated me as a whole person, not just a list of ailments, and given me tools to add to the quality of my life in so many more ways than any doctor I have known. Thank you for helping me get well both physically, mentally and spiritually.
R.R., A.I.A.

Praise for Dr. Nalini

Dr. Chilkov is an invaluable resource for creating a plan for health in the midst of the challenges and complexities of cancer diagnosis, cancer treatment and recovery and investing in the health side of the equation.
Dr. Mark Hyman, M.D.
Five New York Times Best Sellers
UltraWellness, UltraMind, UltraMetabolism, The Blood Sugar Solution
Founder, The UltraWellness Center

Dr. Nalini Chilkov is my number one resource for cutting edge cancer info. She is on the leading edge of Integrative Cancer Care. I have sent my closest friends to her.
JJ Virgin, CNS, CHFS
Celebrity Nutrition and Fitness Expert
Best Selling Author, The Virgin Diet

When it comes to Integrative Cancer Care, Nalini Chilkov is my go to person.
Dr. Frank Lipman M.D.
Holistic Physician
Best Selling Author, Total Renewal

Dr. Chilkov's programs are masterful. You will feel empowered by her toolbox of natural medicines, as well as diet and lifestyle guidelines that are at the root of cancer prevention, cancer recovery and a long and healthy life.
Dr. Sara Gottfried, M.D.
New York Times Best Selling Author The Hormone Cure

TABLE OF CONTENTS

Introduction ix
Do you recognize yourself here? xi
32 Ways to OutSmart Cancer - Book by Dr. Chilkov xv

Part I
OutSmart Cancer Healthy Eating 1
Getting Started 3
Smart Tips 5
QuickStart Strategies for Success 7
Why Does It Matter What You Eat? 9
OutSmart Cancer Healthy Eating Essentials 11
OutSmart Cancer Healthy Meals - What's on Your Plate? 17
OutSmart Cancer Healthy Meals - Breakfast 19
OutSmart Cancer Healthy Meals - Serving Sizes 21
OutSmart Cancer Healthy Meals - Sample Menus 23
OutSmart Cancer Healthy Meals - Foods to Avoid 26
OutSmart Cancer Healthy Meals - Optimal Food Choices 27

Part II
OutSmart Cancer Essential Nutrition Super Shakes 31
Why Shakes 33
Shake Basics 35
Sample Super Shake Recipes 39
Extra Support Options for Super Shakes 41

Copyright © 2014 IntegrativeCancerAnswers.com

Part III
OutSmart Cancer Essential Nutritional & Herbal Supplements 43
OutSmart Cancer Daily Life Insurance Plan - Essential Nutrition 47
Your Complete Five Daily Essentials Kit 53
Extra Nutrients for Added Support 55
OutSmart Cancer RoadMaps 57
A Personal Message from Dr. Nalini Chilkov 59
32 Ways to OutSmart Cancer - Book by Dr. Chilkov 63
Join our Facebook Community 65
Special Offer 67

Introduction

Are you worried about living with cancer? About your future?

Are you worried about getting through treatment?

Recovering and getting your life back?

Are you overwhelmed by all of the conflicting information and advice?

Do you want to take control of your health but are not quite certain what to do?

Are you searching for reliable, trustworthy information?

Are you looking for professional science based guidance from a seasoned expert on how to navigate your cancer journey?

Would you take a big exhale if you could find safe, natural, non-toxic ways to survive and thrive and feel really well, energetic and optimistic, knowing you are doing something life giving towards health, not just against disease?

Would you like to be doing something really positive and life giving?

Something that gave you a solid feeling of faith and confidence and real hope for your future?

Would you feel relieved if you just knew what to do? Then you would happily just move forward and do it!

Are you tired? Exhausted? Fatigued?

Would you like to use your energy for your own healing, not for searching for information and treatments?

Would you like to think about a long and healthy life beyond cancer?

Would you like to GET WELL, STAY WELL AND LIVE WELL?

DO YOU RECOGNIZE YOURSELF HERE?

You want a source of reliable trustworthy professional information.

You are **recently diagnosed, overwhelmed and facing a mountain of confusing and conflicting information.** We will help you sort it out so you can make decisions, talk with your doctor and have a toolbox for supporting your health. You need to prepare, build your strength.

You want to know what really makes a difference and what really works to support health, how to feel better and do better during treatment and recovery.

You may be a cancer patient **currently enduring the stress and exhaustion of cancer treatments** and procedures wondering how you will get through this, knowing it must be possible to **feel less fatigue, less uncertainty.**

You want **more support with side effects and more control over your health and well being.** You know it must be possible to eradicate the cancer and at the same time **protect your healthy cells** and that it must be possible to actually **enhance the quality of your life and feel better** and do better, while going through chemotherapy, radiation and hormone treatments - after all, your life is still happening.

You want **a chance to be healthy and well** when your treatment is completed and you come out the other side ready to get on with your life.

You may be **enduring long-term treatment** (that usually means you will live longer!) You want to address **ongoing side effects** and enhance normal healthy function and **improve the quality of your life and your health every day.**

If you are going to be around for a long time, you want to enjoy your life and not live with pain, struggle with sleep and have plenty of energy for life and for living and feel that you are doing all you can to get better, not worse.

You may be **LIVING BEYOND CANCER** as a cancer survivor (we really don't like that word and we hope you will call yourself a thriver not a survivor), who has either recently or long ago completed your treatments.

You are looking to rebuild, restore, rejuvenate and recover.

You want your life and your body back and you want it to be a healthy life full of vitality, not a life about cancer and side effects, but about really living fully and not worrying about "will my cancer come back" all the time.

You want to be resilient and filled with energy, hope and strength and be able to participate fully and freely in your life.

Or perhaps you have a family history or a high risk of cancer, or perhaps you know, that due to the toxic environmental exposures in your life, you and all the rest of us, have risk for cancer and you just want to **do all you can so that you don't get cancer in the first place.**

I fall into the last category. Both of my parents have had five episodes of cancer combined and I don't want that to be my story. I know I am vulnerable and I am doing everything I can to keep my cancer fighting genes turned on, so I don't live out my genetic potential for getting cancer.

Perhaps you are here because your life has been touched by cancer. Perhaps someone close to you is living with cancer or the aftermath of cancer diagnosis and treatment. You are searching for truly practical, effective and valuable ways to help them, to make a difference for someone you love.
You want **peace of mind.**

What is your story? How did you arrive here?
Please do share it with our openhearted, supportive and caring community. They want to hear from you. I want to hear from you!

Sincerely,
Dr. Nalini Chilkov, L.Ac., O.M.D.

32 Ways To OutSmart Cancer - Create A Body In Which Cancer Cannot Thrive

by Dr. Nalini Chilkov
Founder of Integrative Cancer Answers

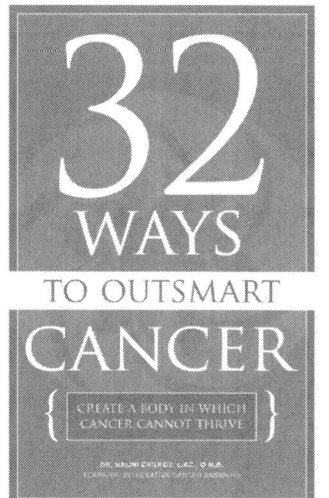

The definitive **step-by-step, easy to follow roadmap** to a cancer free life.

Get access to the same time tested recommendations Dr. Chilkov has made available only to her exclusive celebrity patients for over 30 years.

This **transformational guide** is **for people living with and recovering from cancer and those who do not want to get cancer in the first place**.

Learn how to turn on your cancer fighting genes so that you can live long and live well.

Get Your Copy Now!
http://www.32waysbook.com/

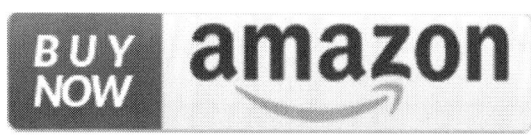

Enjoy Peace of Mind | Feel Confident | Reduce Your Stress
Take Control of Your Health and Your Destiny

Create a Body in which Cancer Cannot Thrive

OUTSMART CANCER
QuickStart GUIDE

Get Answers to Your
Most Common and Most Pressing Questions

WHAT SHOULD I EAT?

WHICH SUPPLEMENTS SHOULD I TAKE?

Included in Your QuickStart Guide

Cancer Fighting Foods Recipes, Meal Plans
Which Foods to Eat
Which Foods To Avoid

The Most Important Immune Enhancing Protective
Nutritional and Herbal Supplements

How to Make Nutritious Delicious Fortifying Protein Super Shakes

Turn on your cancer fighting genes
Choose nourishing protective anti-cancer super foods
Lose Fat Build Muscle
Control inflammation
Promote Healing and Repair

Optimize Immunity and Energy
Protect your cells from damage
Promote longevity and vitality

Copyright © 2014 IntegrativeCancerAnswers.com

PART I

OUTSMART CANCER
HEALTHY EATING

The **BIG** QUESTION everyone asks

What Should I Eat?
What is an Anti-Cancer Diet?
What are the most powerful Cancer Fighting Foods?

And we think you should be ALSO asking

What should I NOT be eating?
Which foods should I avoid
and remove from my diet?

Here is YOUR
LIFE INSURANCE PLAN

**CORE ELEMENTS of YOUR
ANTI CANCER HEALTHY EATING PLAN**

GETTING STARTED

You are about to take the first steps of your own journey to getting well, staying well and living well beyond cancer. You have already taken an important step - you are here! So you have already done much more than most people ever do!

You are about to learn mastery over your own health and longevity. You are about to take control of your destiny.

We are here to show you how to set yourself up to succeed. Allow yourself to be human and to learn gradually, to falter, to get up and dust yourself off and to try again, until you have built a new body and a new life, rooted in supporting your own vitality and health for years to come.

In the same way that you might prepare and build the soil in your garden so that you grow beautiful healthy plants instead of weeds, you are going to transform the inner environment of your own body, so that you grow healthy cells instead of unhealthy cancer cells.

As you read each chapter, stop and review, and make an action plan. Take one step at a time and choose to make changes that feel reasonable and doable. Choose a step that you feel you can accomplish. Make it small. Take that step. Sustain that change. Then pick another step.

Once you have taken just a few steps, made a few changes, the improvement in your quality of life and in your well-being will be palpable to you. You will experience the difference for yourself. All it takes is your participation!

And we at Integrative Cancer Answers and the OutSmart Cancer team are here to support you along the way. Reach out to our community and we will answer your questions. You may find that you want to learn even more and make even more steps once you experience more energy, more clarity, more vitality and are feeling strong and resilient.

The Outsmart Cancer System will take you deeper and deeper and continue to supply you with up to date information and tools for health, longevity and exceptional levels of performance.

Our in depth OutSmart Cancer strategies will continue to show you how to control all of the factors essential to creating a body in which cancer cannot thrive, so that you can live a long and healthy life well beyond cancer and know that you are doing absolutely everything possible.

This OutSmart Cancer QuickStart Guide will put you on solid ground and give you a glimpse of what is really possible for you!

Get ready to get well, stay well and live well beyond cancer!

SMART TIPS

If healthy eating is new for you, start slowly with our **QUICK START STRATEGIES** listed at the end of this section.

Take it slowly. Transform your food choices at a pace that works for you, perhaps over 4-8 weeks.

Yes we know that SOME of you are quantum leapers, ready to jump right in and make sweeping changes. And we also know that MOST of you go in steps and take time to let it all sink in and unfold. And we know that both quantum leapers and one step at a timers will all get to the destination. Each according to your own nature and your own learning style.
The goal here is a long healthy life.

So let's go!

We expect you will be surprised how quickly you start to feel a difference. Each step has its own rewards!

If you already have a lifestyle that includes healthy eating, you may find that you have some fine-tuning and some adjustments to make to refine your anti-cancer food choices and habits. This should be a lot of fun for you, jumping to the next level.

<u>Wherever you are starting:</u> approach one element at a time, integrate a new habit, new pattern, new routine, new food choices that you feel you can do realistically. Take steps, succeed at each step. Be reasonable with yourself. Then go to the next step. Be open, be curious, be willing to experiment. Be willing to be surprised.

After all this is all about YOU thriving. It better be good!

<u>If you need the help of a nutrition or food coach,</u> a nutritionist, or a friend or family member, reach out for the help and support that you need. It is always easier with a buddy, with structure and with guidance.

We invite you to join our community and reach out for support to people just like you. There is nothing like doing it together and sharing with people who are dealing with similar feelings, challenges and wins.

QUICK START Strategies for Success

Pick ONE Starting Point. Make It reasonable!

Start by eating a healthier breakfast for a week.
Next move on to solving lunch, then move on to solving dinner. Then move on to solving what to eat at a restaurant or on an airplane. In one month, you will have made significant changes and you will feel more energetic and have the taste of the quality of well being that you are building and this will become easier and easier and more enjoyable and you will be motivated and inspired to continue!

Start by making breakfast a nutrient dense shake.
Try Our SHAKE IT UP! Super Shake.

Start by cutting out concentrated sweets and sugars and artificial sweeteners for the first week.
Trust me, your taste buds will change and over time the natural sweetness of food will be there and your cravings will decrease because you will have a more normal physiology.

Start by getting rid of all the unhealthy foods in your kitchen at home or at work. Make a Clean Sweep. Out with the bad.

Start by stocking your kitchen and pantry with healthy foods.
Take our FREE OUTSMART CANCER HEALTHY LIVING SHOPPING LIST with you. And in with the good!

Start by going gluten free.

Avoid all wheat, wheat products, oats, barley and rye. Acceptable gluten free and gliadin free grains in moderation, or not all if you are limiting carbohydrates: rice, buckwheat, quinoa, millet.

You will experience a shift in weight, inflammation, swelling, puffiness, mood, bloating, headache, irritability and sleep, if you are very sensitive to these inflammatory grain proteins.

Why Does It Matter What You Eat?

What you choose to eat everyday has a profound influence on health and disease.

You Can Create An Environment That Promotes Healthy Cells and Discourages Cancer Cells.

Depending upon the composition and health of the soil in your garden, you can grow weeds or beautiful healthy plants. In the same way, the environment inside your body surrounding your cells is just like soil in your garden, the nutrients or toxins that are there will determine if you grow cancer cells or healthy cells. That is why it matters what you eat. Let's not grow weeds and cancer cells. Let's build soil that grows beautiful flowers and an inner physiology that supports healthy cells and discourages cancer cells!

Your Food is Information Sending Signals That Turn Your Immune Function On and Off.

Your Food is Literally Talking to Your DNA.

The elements in your food are sending signals to your cells, **turning on protective cancer fighting genes OR turning on deadly cancer promoting genes**, fueling or cooling the fires of inflammation, transforming your blood sugar, body fat, immunity and hormones, creating an environment that can promote health or disease.

We Have Delicious Recipes To Get You Started.

As you discover the power of food to create an Anti-Cancer microenvironment within your body, you will want to start adding these foods to your diet right away.

Our LIVE WELL BLOG on IntegrativeCancerAnswers.com is filled with free, super easy, super healthy, superfood cancer fighting recipes to get you started.

You Can Create a Body in Which Cancer Cannot Thrive!

By making conscious healthy choices every day, you can choose foods that transform your health and contribute to creating a body in which cancer will not thrive.

Bon Appetit!
To Your Long Life and Vibrant Health!

OUTSMART CANCER
HEALTHY EATING ESSENTIALS

EAT ORGANIC, FRESH, WHOLE, UNPROCESSED FOODS FREE OF CHEMICAL AND HORMONE ADDITIVES

Include Foods That Are:

- ✓ Free of artificial colors and flavorings
- ✓ Free of preservatives, herbicides, pesticides, fungicides, sulfites
- ✓ Kick the Packaged Foods and Fast Foods Chains Habits
- ✓ Not Genetically Modified (non GMO)
- ✓ Wild Caught (not farmed raised) Fish
- ✓ Free Range, Grass Fed (not grain fed) meats and poultry
- ✓ High Omega Three Eggs (from free range chickens - look for the dark yellow yolks)
- ✓ Read Labels-Know what is in your food
- ✓ Start Shopping Healthy

Tip: Go to your local health food store or farmers market and ask someone on staff to shop with you, help you find healthy alternatives to your favorite foods, show you all the great choices you have. Notice how much yummy food there is to eat!

EAT AT LEAST 6-8 SERVINGS OF NON STARCHY MULTICOLORED VEGETABLES AND LOW GLYCEMIC FRUITS DAILY

- ✓ 2/3 vegetables and 1/3 fruit (primarily berries)
- ✓ 2/3 of your plate at lunch and dinner should be non-starchy vegetables

Plan on two to three servings per meal of deeply colored fresh plant foods! These foods are rich in anti-oxidants and plant chemicals and healthy fiber.

If you are unable to get your 6-8 servings in every day, supplement with a heaping teaspoon of concentrated GREENS POWDER and/or REDS POWDER and some Fiber Powder in water once or twice daily.

You can put the Greens or Red Powders in your morning shake or in your drinking water, it tastes great!

KICK THE SUGAR HABIT, EAT A LOW GLYCEMIC DIET
to keep your blood sugar and insulin levels normal. Elevated blood sugar and insulin can promote cancer growth.

What is a Low Glycemic Diet?

Avoid all refined sugars and sweeteners. Limit carbohydrates and starches. Read labels. Be aware of hidden sugars in packaged foods. Avoid high glycemic tropical fruits. Choose low glycemic anti-oxidant rich berries. Realize that alcohol is a sugar too!

AVOID: high fructose corn syrup, refined sugars, white sugar, brown sugar, sugar syrups, artificial sweeteners.

Use very sparingly or not at all: honey, maple syrup, black strap molasses, agave, brown rice syrup.

Why is it important?
If you have diabetes, pre diabetes, metabolic syndrome or insulin resistance, struggle with weight loss and fat loss, your diet and/or

genetics may be pre-disposing you to health problems, including cancer.

Stevia, xylitol and maltilol are safe sweeteners and sugar substitutes.

EAT OR DRINK A PROTEIN RICH POWER BREAKFAST EVERY MORNING.

Start the day with a nutrient dense high protein low carb SHAKE IT UP! Daily Kickstart Shake for breakfast. Never Skip Breakfast!

EAT CLEAN LEAN PROTEIN EVERY DAY.

Whether you are an omnivore, a pescaterian, a lacto-ovo vegetarian, a vegan or a Paleo diet fan, you need plenty of protein daily.

- Consume 60-80 grams of high quality protein daily.
- Your morning shake can contain 35-40 grams of protein.
- Each meal should contain at least 20-30 grams (4-5 oz.) of protein.
- Choose from whey or pea protein powder, wild caught fish, grass fed free-range beef, lamb, bison, hormone free eggs, dairy, legumes, or small amounts of nuts and seeds.

What Do I Put in My Shake?
See Instructions for our SHAKE IT UP! Super Shake for guidelines and ideas on page 39 through 41 of this guide.

What Do I Eat for a Power Breakfast If I Don't Have a Shake?
See OUTSMART CANCER HEALTHY MEALS for solutions and ideas on page 27 through 29 of this guide.

EAT AN ANTI-INFLAMMATORY DIET

Avoid high omega six grain fed animal proteins, saturated fats and oils, canola oil, corn oil, rancid oils and foods, excess animal proteins. Eat an abundance of plant-sourced foods.

GO GLUTEN FREE. AVOID GRAINS CONTAINING GLUTEN AND GLIADIN proteins, which may cause inflammatory reactions in the digestive tract and nervous and immune systems.

Avoid wheat and wheat products, oats and oatmeal, barley and rye. Beware of hidden wheat in many foods. Read labels.

You may include these Gluten & Gliadin free whole grains:

- ✓ Quinoa
- ✓ Millet
- ✓ Buckwheat
- ✓ Brown Rice
- ✓ Wild Rice

Try Gluten Free Crackers made from rice or from seeds.

Try almond flour and coconut flour.

While corn is a non-gluten grain, many people have corn sensitivities and should not include corn and corn products in their diet.

Check with your health care provider regarding your food sensitivities and identify which foods may be problematic and inflammatory for you.

Drink Your Daily Required Fluid Intake Every Day.

Drink pure water (filtered or spring), green or herbal teas, soup broths, green drinks (no sweetener), unsweetened coconut water. Fluids are crucial to the health of every organ. Even a little bit of dehydration takes a toll on your health and well being.

How Much?

Your daily requirement for fluids is equal to **half of your body weight in ounces**.

If you weigh 160 pounds you must drink 80 ounces (160 divided by 2) minimum each day. Eight ounces is one full cup and usually one tall drinking glass in the U.S.

SMART TIPS

Get two or three one-quart glass water bottles. Fill them with pure spring water or clean filtered water every morning. Make sure you have consumed all of the water in the bottles by the end of the day. One quart is 32 ounces. Two quarts is 64 ounces.

You can use the water you measured out to make tea or soup or add it to your shake.

Coffee, caffeinated beverages, alcohol and soft drinks, especially those with artificial sweeteners or high fructose corn syrup, do not count towards your daily fluid intake. They either cause fluid loss by increasing urination or actually increase your thirst, rather than quench it.

You can count the fluids consumed in soup, herbal tea, water, green drinks and shakes towards your daily goal.

Remember, this is a MINIMUM daily requirement.

If you live in a hot dry climate, sweat or urinate a lot due to hormonal imbalances, stress or drug side effects, or are engaging in strenuous exercise and physical activity, or are taking chemotherapy drugs - you may need more fluid.

If you have heart, kidney or thyroid disease your doctor may have different recommendations. Consult with your physician, health care provider or a professional nutritionist about the amount of daily fluid intake that is right for you.

KICK THE CAFFEINE HABIT.

While coffee and black tea are all filled with super antioxidants and plant chemicals that are very beneficial, too much caffeine can be a problem, especially if you are tired and wired, under a lot of stress or having difficulty sleeping restfully.

If you do drink coffee or black tea, make sure they are organic. Coffee in particular is one of the most heavily sprayed pesticide contaminated crops. Limit yourself to one cup in the morning.

Green tea does have a small amount of caffeine, but it is not a problem for most people. If you are a caffeine sensitive person, you probably know that you won't be able to sleep if you have a cup of tea or coffee, or even chocolate after 4PM!

Listen to your body!

OUTSMART CANCER HEALTHY MEALS

WHAT'S ON YOUR PLATE?

A little less than half of your plate is non-starchy green leafy and deeply colored vegetables

¼ of your plate is clean healthy protein

¼ of your plate is healthy fats and oils

1/8 of your plate is high fiber carbohydrates and low glycemic index fruits
(mostly berries)

1/8 of your plate is a combination of hormone free dairy products or fresh organic nuts and seeds

A little organic dark chocolate or organic sulfite free red wine

EAT FRESH WHOLE ORGANIC UNPROCESSED CHEMICAL FREE FOOD!

Your Food Should Be:

Free Range, Grass Fed
Hormone Free Wild (NOT Farm Raised) Fish
Organic
Pesticide Free
Herbicide Free
Preservative Free
No Artificial Flavorings or Colorings

NO Blackened, Grilled or Smoked Food
NO Heating OR Storing Food in Plastic or Styrofoam

EAT REAL FOOD!
If you cannot pronounce it - don't eat it!

OUTSMART CANCER HEALTHY MEALS

BREAKFAST

1-2 servings of Clean Healthy Protein (approximately 20-40 grams)
1-3 servings of Healthy Fats and Oils
1-2 servings of Starches or High Fiber Low Glycemic Carbohydrates
2 servings of non-starchy Vegetables

OR

SHAKE IT UP! Super Shake
High in protein, fiber and antioxidants
Feel free to have more than one shake a day!

LUNCH AND DINNER

1 serving of Clean Healthy Protein (approximately 20 grams or 4 ounces)
1-3 servings of Healthy Fats and Oils
2-4 servings of Non Starchy Low Glycemic Green & Deeply Colorful ORGANIC Vegetables

OPTIONAL HEALTHY DESSERT

Low glycemic Organic fresh fruit (especially berries), Organic Un-sulphured dried fruit, 80% Dark Chocolate

SMART TIP

You can enjoy a SHAKE as a meal substitute
or as a source of extra protein, fiber and nutrients.

OUTSMART CANCER HEALTHY MEALS SERVING SIZES

PROTEIN SERVINGS

We recommend **60-80 grams total daily protein** or 3-4 20 gram servings daily.

20 grams of protein = 3-4 oz cooked chicken, fish, beef, lamb or bison
1 medium high omega three egg = 5 grams of protein

4 oz (1/2 Cup) Organic Hormone Free Cottage Cheese or Greek Yoghurt = 15-20 grams protein
2 tablespoons of almond butter = 10 grams protein

1 cup (8oz) cooked beans = 15 grams protein
or 1 large bowl of bean soup = 15 grams protein
or 6 ounces of Firm Tofu or Tempeh

1 heaping tablespoon whey protein powder (1 scoop of Whey Cool) or
2 heaping tablespoons pea (Pure Pea Protein Powder) or rice protein powder
20-22 grams protein

HEALTHY FATS AND OILS

1 serving
1 tablespoon of olive oil, coconut oil, ghee
¼ avocado

1 tablespoon of nut butter
10-12 nuts
5-6 olives
4 ounces of cold water fish such as wild salmon, cod, mackerel or sardines

GREEN LEAFY AND DEEPLY COLORED LOW STARCH LOW GLYCEMIC VEGETABLES AND BERRIES

1 serving = ½ cup cooked or 1 cup raw

HIGH FIBER STARCHY MODERATE GLYCEMIC CARBOHYDRATES

1 serving
½ cup cooked beans or whole grains
1 slice of whole grain gluten free bread
1 piece of fruit OR 1 oz. 70+% organic dark chocolate

OUTSMART CANCER HEALTHY MEALS SAMPLE MENUS

LOW GLYCEMIC GLUTEN FREE ANTIOXIDANT RICH

SAMPLE MENU 1

Green and multicolored salad with sprouts, extra virgin olive oil, basil, and squeezed lemon or lime

Baked cod topped with avocado salsa
Chop 1 avocado, 1 tomato, ½ c. red onion, ½ c. capers (drained), 1/4 c. fresh cilantro, ½ tsp. cumin, 1/8 tsp. cayenne and 2 tbsp. lime juice

½ cup cooked quinoa

SAMPLE MENU 2

Large mixed green and multicolored salad with non-starchy veggies of your choice

Grilled chicken or fish, topped with extra virgin olive oil, lemon, and herbs of your choice

SAMPLE MENU 3

Chicken salad (made with olive oil) wrapped in a large lettuce leaf. Feel free to add grated carrots, avocado, or other veggies of your choice.

SAMPLE MENU 4

Organic vegetable broth

Shrimp and vegetables: sauté fresh tail-on shrimp and chopped garlic
(Roughly chop 10 different vegetables and lightly stir-fry with freshly grated ginger, lightly drizzle sesame oil in a non-stick ceramic pan)

½ cup cooked buckwheat noodles

SAMPLE MENU 5

Baby greens salad with extra virgin olive oil and squeezed lemon or lime

Grilled buffalo burger on a Portabella mushroom

Mixed roasted vegetables: roast combination of cauliflower, broccoli, Brussels sprouts, onions and squash in extra virgin olive oil and herbs to taste (turmeric, basil or rosemary)

OUTSMART CANCER HEALTHY MEALS

FOODS TO AVOID

AVOID Concentrated Sweets and Sugars
Including sucrose, fructose, high fructose corn syrup, honey, and maple syrup.

AVOID Artificial Sweeteners
Sucralose, maltodextrin, saccharin, aspartame, Sweet 'n' Low, Splenda, Equal.

ACCEPTABLE Sweeteners
Natural low-impact sweeteners such as stevia and polyols, xylitol and erythritol, and dried fruit are allowed.

AVOID Gluten and Gliadin-containing Grains
Avoid foods that contain wheat, oats, rye, spelt, kamut, bulgur, couscous, and barley. This includes pastas, bread, crackers, cereals, and other products made with or from these grains.

PERMITTED Grains
You CAN include Safe Gluten-free whole grains such as brown rice, wild rice, millet, quinoa, amaranth, and buckwheat.

AVOID Cows Milk Dairy Products
Including milk, cheese, yogurt and ice cream especially if you have allergies and sensitivities.

PERMITTED Dairy Products
Try goat or sheep's milk, coconut milk, almond milk, hemp milk.

AVOID All Alcohol and Caffeine-containing Beverages
Including coffee, tea and soda.

AVOID Soy Protein
Including tofu and tempeh, if you are allergic or sensitive to soy.

AVOID Sugary Unhealthy Desserts
Candy, cakes, cookies, ice cream.

AVOID Processed, Packaged Foods

AVOID Fried Foods, Hydrogenated Oils, Margarine

AVOID Peanuts/Peanut Butter (highly allergenic)

OUTSMART CANCER HEALTHY MEALS
OPTIMAL FOOD CHOICES

OPTIMAL PROTEIN CHOICES

Organic/Hormone-Free Chicken, Turkey, Lamb and Beef	Cold Water Fish - salmon, halibut, cod, mackerel, tuna - choose wild ocean fish over farm raised fish
Wild game	Organic Eggs
Organic legumes	

OPTIMAL HEALTHY FATS AND OILS CHOICES

Flaxseed Oil	Walnut Oil
Extra Virgin Olive Oil	Organic Coconut Oil
Hempseed	Avocado
Raw Nuts	Organic Cultured Butter
Raw Seeds	Ghee

OPTIMAL FRUIT CHOICES

Blueberries	Strawberries
Raspberries	Blackberries
Cranberries	

OPTIMAL NON-STARCHY VEGETABLE CHOICES

Arugula	Radishes	Onions
Asparagus	Cucumber	Parsley
Bamboo shoots	Dandelion greens	

Copyright © 2014 IntegrativeCancerAnswers.com

Bean sprouts	Eggplant	Radicchio
Beet greens	Endives	Snap beans
Bell peppers (yellow, red, green)	Fennel	Snap peas
Broad beans	Garlic	Shallots
Broccoli	Ginger Root	Spinach
Brussels sprouts	Green beans	Spaghetti squash
Cabbage	Hearts of Palm	Summer squash
Cassava	Jicama	Swiss chard
Cauliflower	Jalapeno peppers	Tomatoes
Celery	Kale	Turnip greens
Chicory	Kohlrabi	Watercress
Chives	Lettuce	
Collard Greens	Mustard Greens	

HIGH FIBER STARCHY CARBOHYDRATE CHOICES

Artichokes	Turnip	Great northern beans
Squash (acorn, winter, butter)	Legumes	Kidney beans
Leaks	Black beans	Lentils
Lima beans	Adzuki beans	Mung beans
Okra	Buckwheat	Navy beans
Pumpkin	Chickpeas	Pinto beans
Sweet potato or yams	Cowpeas	Split peas
Yellow beans	French beans	White beans

MODERATE GLYCEMIC INDEX FRUIT CHOICES

Eat sparingly, or after a workout:

Cherries	Plums	Prunes
Pears	Oranges	Apples
Apricots	Peaches	Kiwi fruit
Melons	Grapefruits	Nectarines
Tangerines		

HERBS AND SPICES

All herbs and spices are rich in antioxidants and many contain potent anti-cancer compounds:

Garlic	Sage	Chili peppers
Ginger	Curcumin	Coriander
Oregano	Cinnamon	Cumin
Rosemary	Saffron	Cardamom
Thyme	Black Pepper	

PART II

OUTSMART CANCER

ESSENTIAL NUTRITION

SUPER SHAKES

BUILD YOUR FOUNDATION OF STRENGTH AND IMMUNITY

FORTIFY WITH PROTEIN EVERY DAY

We recommend 60-80 grams of protein daily!

SHAKE IT UP!

SUPER SHAKES

Include at least one shake daily, preferably for breakfast. You can use additional shakes to supplement your protein, fiber and nutrients if needed.

Why Shakes

When you create a high protein, high fiber, super antioxidant shake and drink one or two servings daily, you will be feeding your cells optimum levels of nutrients and creating a high level of health and well being.

You will be optimizing your nutrition, getting more nutrients in one serving than at most meals.

- ✓ You will be building muscle and burning fat and creating a lean, healthy body
- ✓ You will be supplying the building blocks for sustained energy, endurance and stamina
- ✓ You will be alert, sharp and thinking clearly, perhaps even brilliantly

- ✓ You will be promoting normal control of inflammation and immunity
- ✓ You will be filling your body with nature's own cell protective super antioxidants

And we think you just may have a bit more sparkle in your eye and bounce in your step!

Do I have to have my shake in the morning for breakfast?

If you prefer a WARM breakfast, have your shake later in the day.

See sample meals and menus on page 23 through 29 of this guide.

What About Other Sources of Protein?

See page 27 for suggestions.

SHAKE BASICS

A Beginner's Guide to Making a Super Shake

1. Choose a Protein
>Whey Protein (contains cows milk dairy protein fraction) or Pea Protein (vegan and dairy free)

2. Choose a Fiber
>Paleo Fiber or
>High Lignan Flax Seed Meal

3. Choose a Fruit or Vegetable or Concentrate
Organic Low Glycemic Fruits are preferred to keep your blood sugar and insulin metabolism normal. This is protective to your cells, but also supports sustained energy, fat burning and muscle building.

Ideal Fruits
Organic fresh or frozen berries (low glycemic and high in cell protective plant chemicals due to their COLOR).

Avocado: adds monounsaturated healthy fats and makes your shake more creamy.

Avoid tropical fruits or use sparingly. Tropical fruits are more sugary, more glycemic. Tropical fruits tend to be very heavily sprayed with insecticides and anti-fungal chemicals. These include banana, papaya, mango, and pineapple.

Ideal Vegetables
Spinach, Kale, Chard, Parsley, Celery, Cucumber

4. Choose a Liquid

Filtered Water, Unsweetened Coconut Water, Coconut Milk or Almond Milk are the best choices.

5. Choose SHAKE Extras (Optional)

Get Creative
Think about adding fresh or dried herbs and spices (about ½ teaspoon per serving).

Fresh Mint adds a refreshing dimension.
Fresh or Dried Ginger Root adds a spicy warmth.
Cinnamon Powder adds a sweet spicy flavor.
Vanilla extract makes you feel royal and rich.

All of the above add flavor due to their essential oils, which also support normal digestive function.

Turmeric has a beautiful golden color, does not have a strong taste (you won't really notice that it's there) and adds support for normal inflammation control and normal regulation of cell cycling, making it one of the top cancer fighting spices.

Refer to the EXTRA SUPPORT section below for additional nutrients and herbs to make your shake a truly healing tonic.

Place all ingredients in your blender or shaker bottle and SHAKE IT UP! Blend until smooth. (That's why we call it a smoothie!)

DRINK UP!

Professional Quality, Doctor Recommended Supplements
Pure Body Systems | Simply Superior Supplements
www.purebodysystems.com

SAMPLE SUPER SHAKE RECIPES

Basic Super Shake

2 scoops of Whey Cool (Vanilla or unflavored) OR Pure Pea Dairy Free (Vanilla or Unflavored)
1 Tablespoon of PaleoFiber
1-2 teaspoons of PaleoGreens and/or PaleoReds
1/2 cup of frozen organic berries
1/2 cup of water or coconut milk, almond milk, cashew milk

Blend with ice to make a thicker shake

Berry Cherry Antioxidant Shake

1 scoop Whey Cool, Pure Pea Protein (Dairy Free) or Paleo Cleanse (Dairy Free)
1 Scoop Paleo Meal or Paleo Meal Dairy Free
1 teaspoon PaleoFiber
2 teaspoons PaleoGreens
1 cup frozen blackberries or blueberries
1 cup frozen cherries (optional)
1 cup almond or coconut milk
1 teaspoon freshly grated nutmeg

Green and Gold Healing Smoothie

2 scoops Whey Cool Vanilla or Pure Pea Vanilla Protein (Dairy Free)
2 tablespoons PaleoGreens

1 tablespoon flaxseed meal or chia seeds OR 2 teaspoons PaleoFiber
½ teaspoon turmeric powder
1 cup coconut milk

Maca Power Shake

1 scoop Paleo Meal Vanilla or Paleo Meal Vanilla Dairy Free
1 scoop Whey Cool Vanilla or Pure Pea Vanilla Dairy Free
1 cup unsweetened coconut milk
½ cup water
½ avocado
2 dates
1 tablespoon maca powder
¼ teaspoon cinnamon
2 cups fresh spinach or kale leaves

Additions for SHAKE IT UP! Super Shakes
EXTRA SUPPORT OPTIONS

Extra Cell Protective Antioxidants
Paleo Greens Organic Powder 1 heaping teaspoon
Paleo Reds Berry Powder 1 heaping teaspoon

Extra Energy and Muscle Support
Carnitine Tartrate Powder ½ teaspoon

Extra Brain and Nervous System Support
Brain Vitale Powder ½ teaspoon
Phosphatidyl Choline granules 1 tablespoon

Extra Digestive and Immune System Support
Probiotic Synergy Powder ¼ teaspoon

Extra Strength, Stamina and Resilience
Maca Powder 1/2 - 1 teaspoon
Cordyceps Powder 1/2 teaspoon
Coriolus Powder 1/2 teaspoon

PART III

OUTSMART CANCER

ESSENTIAL NUTRITIONAL & HERBAL SUPPLEMENTS

OUTSMART CANCER
ESSENTIAL NUTRITIONAL & HERBAL SUPPLEMENTS

INCLUDE ESSENTIAL SUPPORTIVE NUTRITIONAL SUPPLEMENTS EVERY DAY. This is the CORE of your long-term foundation for health.

Feeding your cells OPTIMAL levels of nutrients, rather than MINIMUM daily requirements may transform your health.

During times of stress, with the challenges of surgery, chemotherapy and radiation there is a higher need for nutrients.

For recovery, restoration and revitalization and to build vibrant health and longevity, include essential nutritional and herbal supplements.

The inclusion of super nutritious shakes filled with protein, fiber and antioxidant foods is the key to robust immunity, sustainable energy, increased resistance and the capacity to heal and repair; the foundation of resilience and wellness.

At a MINIMUM take your **FIVE ESSENTIAL NUTRIENTS AND YOUR SUPER SHAKE EVERY DAY**

QUICK START STEP

Start taking the FIVE ESSENTIAL DAILY SUPPLEMENTS everyday.

Be consistent. You will feel the difference.

Take one dose twice daily with food in your stomach.

OR spread out your supplements into three or four smaller doses over the course of the day if you wish. Just get the full DAILY dose.

Be PRACTICAL and DO WHAT WORKS FOR YOU!

SMART TIP

It is very easy to take your morning dose of vitamins with your SHAKE IT UP! Morning Breakfast Super Shake or with your breakfast!

Take your second dose with Lunch or Dinner with food in your stomach.

Caution:
Talk to Your Doctor If You Take Thyroid Medication.
Calcium may interfere with the absorption of thyroid medications.
If you take Thyroid medication, many physicians recommend that you take your thyroid medication on an empty stomach when you wake up and wait one hour after taking your thyroid medication, before taking your calcium supplements. Caffeine also interferes with thyroid medication.

THIS IS YOUR LIFE INSURANCE PLAN

OUTSMART CANCER ESSENTIAL FOUNDATION NUTRITION
for Mastering Vibrant Health and Longevity

**YOUR EVERY DAY
HEALTHY LIVING PRESCRIPTION**

**FIVE DAILY ESSENTIAL NUTRIENTS
AND
DAILY SHAKE IT UP! SUPER SHAKE**

OUTSMART CANCER
DAILY LIFE INSURANCE PLAN
ESSENTIAL NUTRITION

FIVE DAILY ESSENTIAL NUTRIENTS

Optional: capsules can be opened up and the contents added to your shake.

1. Copper Free Iron Free Metabolic Maintenance Multi Vitamin

Recommended: Metabolic Synergy™
High Potency Optimized Formula with added Cell Protection and Blood Sugar Stabilizing Support
Recommended dose: 3 capsules 2x/day

Rich in the immune supporting and anti-aging antioxidants such as Vitamin C, D, E, and lipoic acid, while also providing B-complex, Pantothenic Acid and highly absorbable forms of true chelate minerals including **calcium**, magnesium, potassium, **balanced iodine and selenium along with** chromium, vanadium, manganese, **boron, biotin and zinc.**

The following nutrients are included in this amazing formula:
600 mg lipoic acid + 4 mg biotin - prevents the typical reduction in carboxylase enzymes seen in research when lipoic acid is given alone. These two nutrients together aid healthy insulin secretion and glucose metabolism
- ✓ *600 mg taurine, 100mg EGCg from green tea and 400 IU vitamin D* - all of which help insulin to work better

- ✓ *50 mg benfothiamine, 200 mg carnosine and 100 IU of high gamma vitamin E* - to protect from neuropathy & kidney damage
- ✓ *3000 IU vitamin A* - important for immune system
- ✓ *25 mg vitamin B1 (as thiamine HCl)* - needed for energy
- ✓ *100 mcg molybdenum* - needed for detoxification

Low Cost Alternative: Twice Daily Multi
Copper Free Iron Free Basic Daily Formula
Recommended dose: 1 capsule 2x/day

This foundation formula covers your basic daily needs, is rich in antioxidants and is great for both men and women. Remember to add Calcium Malate Chelate and Magnesium Malate Chelate separately. However it does not offer all of the added benefits and protections of Metabolic Synergy™ above which we recommend when your goal is to OUTSMART CANCER.

2. EPA DHA OMEGA 3 FATTY ACIDS from Fish Oil with added Vitamin D and Vitamin K (all in one).

Recommended: OmegAvail Ultra™ + Vitamin D & Vitamin K
Recommended dose: 2 capsules 2x/day

This product contains a very pure, highly bioavailable and stable form of these essential for life oils. Each 2 capsules contain 1000 mg of Omega 3 oils and 1000 units of Vitamin D3. Your daily dose of 2 caps twice daily provides 2000mg of EPA plus DHA and 2000 units of Vitamin D3. Optimized doses of Vitamin K1 and K2 are included in this outstanding formula.

Omega 3 oils are essential to normal inflammation control, healthy brain and nervous system function, healthy cell walls and cell communication and signaling. These oils are crucial to normal heart health, immune health and bone and joint health.

Vitamin D is vital to normal immunity, mood, cardiovascular and bone health.

You may wish to ask your doctor to measure your levels of Omega 3 and Omega 6 fats in your blood to be sure you have the correct levels and ratios.

It is also important to monitor and measure blood levels of Vitamin D3 to be sure you are taking the right dose. Many people require customized dosing to achieve optimum immune enhancing levels of Vitamin D3.

Vitamin K is crucial to normal calcium metabolism and bone health as well as enhancing normal immune function.

This is an unusual formula which cuts down the number of pills you have to take because it combines all of these synergistic nutrients in each capsule.

3. Probiotic Supplement supplying active health friendly bacteria

Recommended: Probiotic Synergy™
Recommended dose: 1 capsule 2x/daily

Probiotics are a source of health friendly bacteria vital to normal immunity, normal inflammation control, normal mood balance, normal detoxification function, normal intestinal health and normal hormone metabolism. The impact of these organisms on immunity cannot be overstated.

Be sure to also include healthy fermented foods in your diet on a regular basis to boost your immunity and assure normal digestion and elimination.

Fully Reacted Chelated Minerals in a one to one ratio

We recommend a one to one ratio of calcium and magnesium rather than the two to one ratio found in most supplements. Malates are readily absorbed, enhancing the availability of these essential minerals.

These mineral supplements provide a Copper Free Source of Highly Absorbable Calcium and Magnesium. Be careful when choosing bone support formulas, most of which contain copper. When creating an environment in your body that is not hospitable to cancer low normal copper levels are important. Therefore we do not recommend supplements that contain copper. Normal amounts of copper can be provided by eating a diet rich in vegetables, nuts, seeds, whole grains and beans.

4. Calcium

Recommended: Calcium Malate Chelate
Recommended dose: 1-2 capsules 2x/daily
2 capsules provide 500 mg

Calcium is a critical mineral that functions not only in bone health but also in normalizing blood pressure, blood vessel health, normal sleep and relaxation. Deficiencies have been linked to increased rates of some cancers including colon cancer and pancreatic cancer.

5. Magnesium

Recommended: Magnesium Malate Chelate
Recommended dose: 1-2 capsules 2x/daily
2 capsules provide 500 mg

Magnesium Malate Chelate contains two superior forms of magnesium: one fully chelated to glycine and the other bound to malic acid, which gives this formula excellent absorption and health-promoting properties.

Malic acid is found naturally in apples and other fruits and vegetables. This organic mineral acid complex is included because of malic acid's role in the Krebs cycle, which may help support energy production.

Glycine, which is found in foods and is synthesized by the body, aids in the normal absorption of minerals. Glycine is also of low molecular weight, making it ideal for chelating and absorbing magnesium. The unique properties of this magnesium formula allow for greater absorption and tolerability than non-bound magnesium salts available on the market.

MAKE IT EASY AND SAVE MONEY

Get Your COMPLETE Five Daily Essentials KIT

www.purebodysystems.com/five-daily-essentials-kit-designs-for-health.html

Metabolic Synergy™ : 3 caps twice daily
OmegAvail Ultra™ +Vitamin D : 1 cap twice daily
Probiotic Synergy™ : 1 twice daily
Calcium Malate Chelate : 1-2 caps twice daily
Magnesium Malate Chelate : 1-2 caps twice daily

Professional Quality Doctor Recommended Supplements
Pure Body Systems | Simply Superior Supplements
www.purebodysystems.com

EXTRA NUTRIENTS FOR ADDED SUPPORT

Enhance Vital Energy, Fight Fatigue, Enhance Immunity
Kidney Korrect™ 2 caps twice daily
Hepatatone Plus™ 2 caps twice daily

Herbal Super Cellular Protection
C3 Curcumin 1-2 caps twice daily
Broccoprotect™ Sulphoraphane 1-2 caps twice daily
Resveratrol Synergy™ (Resveratrol plus Quercitin) 1-2 caps twice daily
EGCG GreenTea Extract 1-2 caps twice daily

Nutrient Super Cellular Protection
CoQNol Ubiquinol CoQ10 100mg 1 cap twice daily
Lipoic Acid Supreme 1-2 caps twice daily
N-Acetyl Cysteine 1-2 caps twice daily
Milk Thistle 1-2 caps twice daily

SMART TIP
Capsules can be opened up and the contents added to your daily shake.

Professional Quality Doctor Recommended Supplements
Pure Body Systems | Simply Superior Supplements
www.purebodysystems.com

Copyright © 2014 IntegrativeCancerAnswers.com

OUTSMART CANCER ESSENTIALS GUIDES
GUIDING YOU THROUGH EVERY PHASE OF YOUR JOURNEY

JUST DIAGNOSED ESSENTIALS
PREPARE | STRENGTHEN | FORTIFY

IN TREATMENT ESSENTIALS
PROTECT | NOURISH | SUPPORT

AFTER TREATMENT ESSENTIALS
RECOVER | REBUILD | RESTORE

LIFE BEYOND CANCER ESSENTIALS
MASTERY | HEALTH | VITALITY | LONGEVITY

Download your FREE OutSmart Cancer Essentials Guide at
IntegrativeCancerAnswers.com

A Personal Message from Dr. Nalini Chilkov

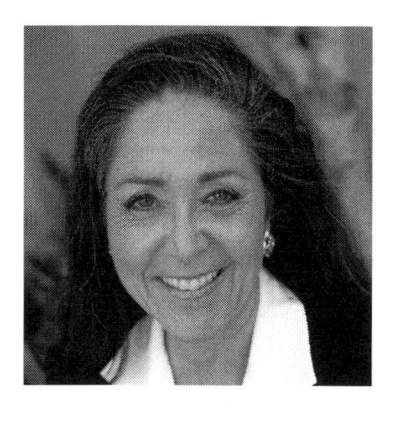

Modern Cancer Care is primarily focused on the disease, on the cancer itself as the enemy.

There is little focus on creating and sustaining real health and usually none on you, the patient as a whole person, a unique individual. Conventional cancer care can be a very cookbook formulaic system of recipes. If you get cancer A, you hope the recipe for Cancer A will work on you and your cancer. Sometimes it does and often it does not.

Individualized care is really what is needed. You need someone to look really deeply into the roots of your illness and into the roots of a long-term solution.

This is what Integrative Cancer Care and the **Outsmart Cancer Programs** are all about. A Healthy YOU. Giving you the tools for health so your life is not focused on cancer but on you, your dreams, your visions, your well being, your health and longevity. What really causes all of that?

With a primary focus on illness alone and on fighting only the cancer you are stuck with a very limited approach.

What about health? What about protecting the healthy cells? What about preserving health and restoring health and making health enduring so that the fear of recurrence is not always lurking and waiting to rear its ugly head? Why do we just wait and watch and hope nothing bad happens again? That is so passive! You can take action. You can do more.

I am on a mission. I am on fire. These questions have become my life's passion. I want to teach you mastery for the health side of your equation.

It is possible to create a body inhospitable to cancer growth and development.

It is possible to create and sustain an anti-cancer environment for your cells that promotes health and resists cancer. All with safe, natural nutritional supplements and herbs, with cancer fighting super foods, with very targeted steps to take you to solid ground where you are not worried about cancer, where you are not plagued by side effects, where you can actually plan for your future.

You can **create an anti-cancer life, a body that supports health and discourages cancer.** It is easy and the better you feel, the more energy you have, the more fun it becomes.

Now, after three decades of experience, all I have learned, all of the programs that have only been available to a very exclusive clientele in my clinic, the same time tested programs are available to you. I believe, actually it is my experience, that **each and every person whose life has been touched by cancer has the potential to get well, stay well and live well beyond cancer.** Build a body in which cancer cannot thrive.

I have developed the in depth OutSmart Cancer Programs for you to show you how to live cancer free and worry free.

This OutSmart Cancer QuickStart Guide is your launching pad - a way to get started right now, right away. A way to start taking action right now on the OutSmart Cancer path to health and longevity - a path to freedom and liberation from the dark cloud of cancer. A path into the brilliant sunlight, where you are living your own vibrant healthy life on your own terms as a result of taking action.

In your OutSmart Cancer Quick Start Guide you will find the first steps that you will take that are gong to make a difference in the rest of your life.

I am so thrilled you are here.

I extend a Warm Welcome to you from the OutSmart Cancer Community!

And I toast Your Long and Healthy Life!

Sincerely
Dr. Nalini Chilkov, L.Ac., O.M.D.

32 Ways To OutSmart Cancer - Create A Body In Which Cancer Cannot Thrive

by Dr. Nalini Chilkov
Founder of Integrative Cancer Answers

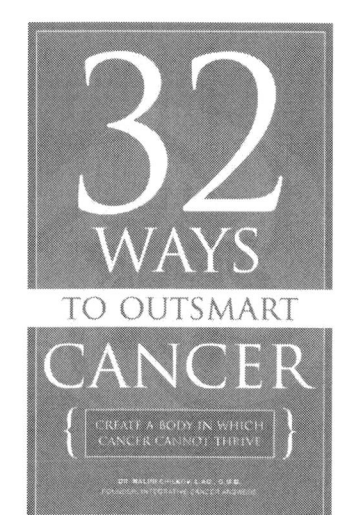

The definitive **step by step easy to follow roadmap** to a cancer free life.

Get access to the same time tested recommendations Dr. Chilkov has made available only to her exclusive celebrity patients for over 30 years.

This **transformational guide** is **for people living with and recovering from cancer and those who do not want to get cancer in the first place**.

Learn how to turn on your cancer fighting genes so that you can live long and live well.

Get Your Copy Now!
http://www.32waysbook.com/

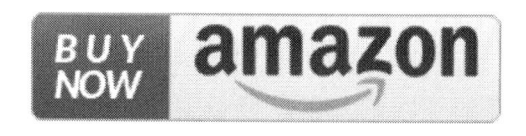

INTEGRATIVE CANCER ANSWERS

Visit the Community - Join the Conversation!

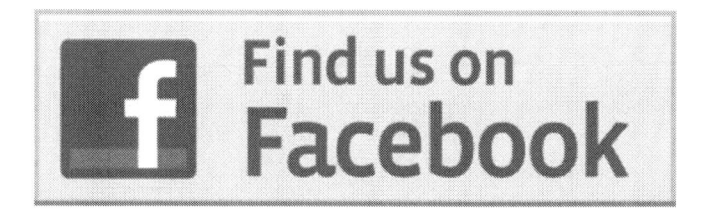

Find us on Facebook

Join us today!

For more resources and tips for Outsmarting Cancer,
visit www.IntegrativeCancerAnswers.com

Special Offer

Our Gift To You.

Get **10% Off Your First Order** for Superior Professional Grade Supplements at our Pure Body Systems Store.

To place your order and claim your discount, go to

www.PureBodySystems.com

and enter your discount code
OUTSMART

For more inspiration, tips and resources for creating vibrant health and longevity,
visit
www.IntegrativeCancerAnswers.com

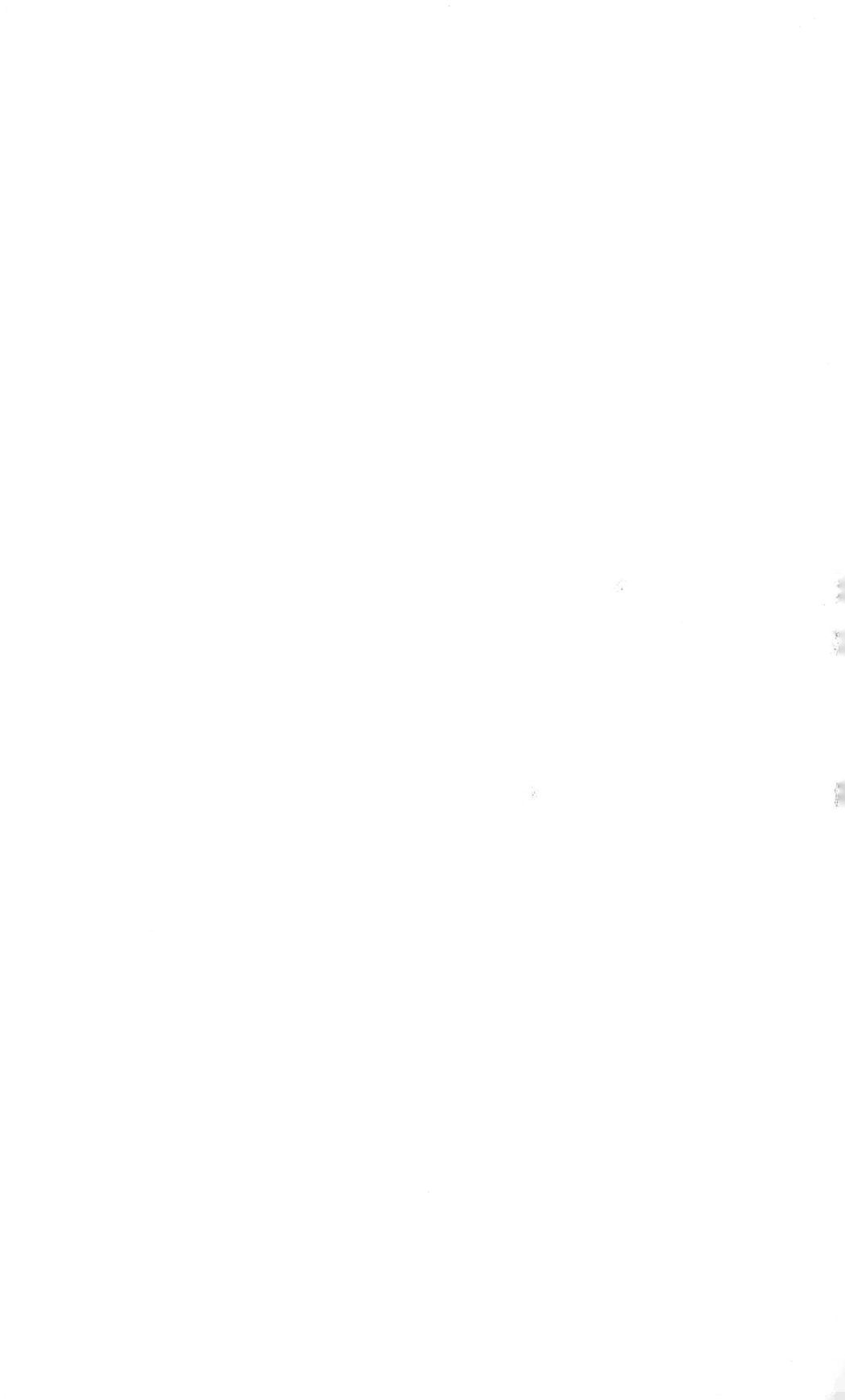

Made in the USA
Middletown, DE
30 May 2021